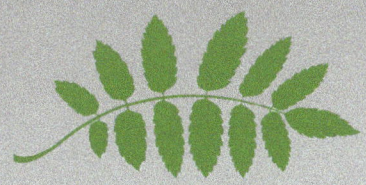

WEST END ORGANIX

Ageless Beauty, Organic Health

Look and feel younger and healthier with our natural remedies products!

www.WestEndOrganix.com

Discount: 10% off of your order - Code *WEO2021*

PUMP IT UP MAGAZINE
LINKS

WEBSITE
www.pumpitupmagazine.com

FACEBOOK
www.facebook.com/pumpitupmagazine

TWITTER
www.twitter.com/pumpitupmag

SOUNDCLOUD
www.soundcloud.com/pumpitupmagazine

INSTAGRAM
pumpitupmagazine

PINTEREST
www.pinterest.com/pumpitupmagazine

PUMP IT UP MAGAZINE
30721 Russell Ranch Road
Suite 140
Westlake Village,
California 91362
United States

 (818)514 – 0038(Ext:102)
 info@pumpitupmagazine.com

Pump it up Magazine

TABLE OF CONTENTS

⚡ **EDITORIAL** 6
Page 5

⚡ **SMILEY J**
THE QUEEN OF TH BEST PODCAST
FOR INDEPENDENT MUSIC ARTISTS

⚡ **BEAUTY - FASHION**
- 8 ways to look after your skin
- Neon green the new trend

⚡ **TOP TIPS** 11
How getting on podcasts
can help your music career

⚡ **WELLNESS**
5 days love yourself challenge

⚡ **QUIZ & GAME**
- Are You Anxious
- Crosswords

⚡ **FITNESS** 18
Slim & Sexy
30 days
body challenge

⚡ **MOVIES**
- Best indie movies
to watch

⚡ **WHAT'S HOT** 22
- How to find a new hobby
as an adult
- Best things to do in L.A.
- How to cook great food
without the hassle

⚡ **HUMANITARIAN AWARENESS**
Hobbies to reduce anxiety

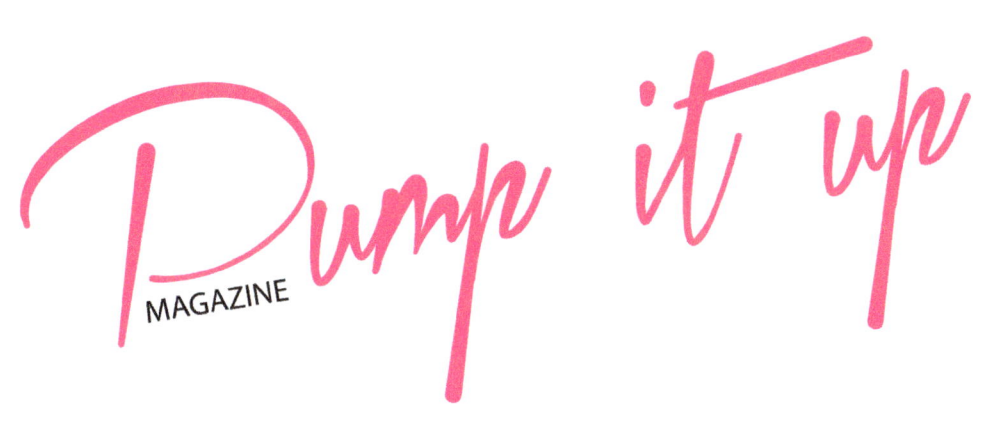

Pump it up
MAGAZINE

EDITORIAL

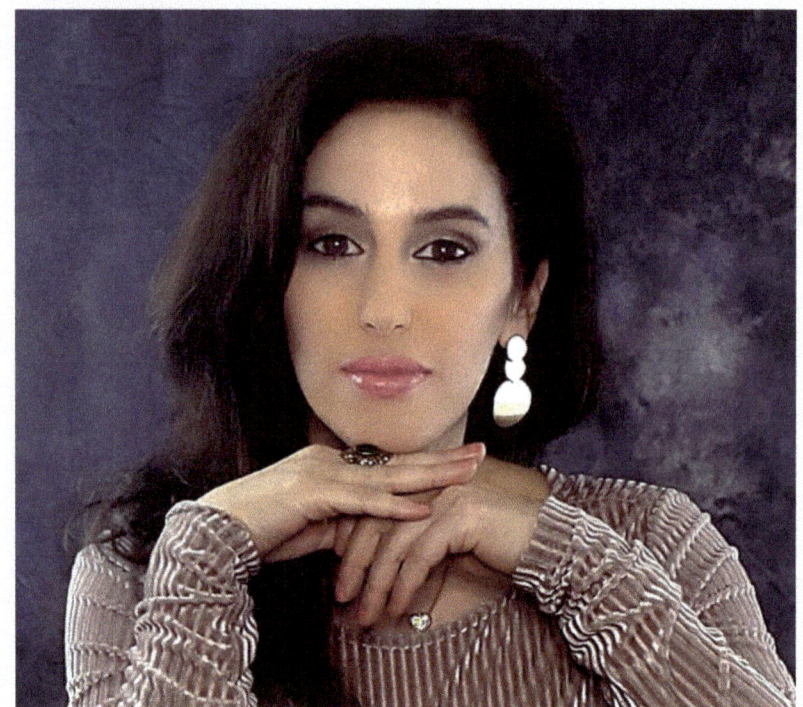

Greetings,

It's warming up here in Southern California and we haven't had much rain,
But I love the warm weather, I'm hoping to hit the beaches soon.
I'm hoping that this months edition of Pump it Up Magazine will warm your hearts and spirits in these challenging times.

On the cover we have podcast queen, Smiley J. Who has interviewed tons of guests on her popular show, The Smiley J. Artist Zone .
I'm personally grateful to have Smiley J. on the cover of or May edition. Her love and support for indie music creators mirrors my mission here at Pump It Up.
Keep up the good work Smiley J. I feel ya girl. We need your spotlight to continue to shine on the indie music creator.
Keep reading and final put more about
how being on podcasts can boost your music career.

Can you all feel the mental signs of the times. There is so much info to take in. The good, the bad , and the ugly. One therapist said , "I've had to work with more anxiety patients than I ever had to. "

We've got some fun games in this issue and some little gems to take a load off.
If you're bored and want to tune out the negative , then tune in to KPIU-DB radio for some great music . From hip hop to Jazz, we've got something for you.
By the way, my good friend Bernie Capodici, has a great and informative book out.
It's called Modern Recording Artist Handbook.
Got questions about the industry? Order a copy today.

Hope you've been exercising and eating healthy. I'm love my veggies
and my vegan croissants!
My hubby Michael loves my Sweet Potato pies. He doesn't have to wait till the holidays but is the humble recipient of two every few weeks .

Well that's all for now
May God bless you!
Remember , the answer to a linear life is to become creative!

Anissa Sutton

CONTRIBUTORS

FOUNDER
Anissa Sutton

EDITOR
Michael B. Sutton

FASHION
Tiffani Sutton

MARKETING
Grace Rose
Carter Kaya

PARTNERS

Editions L.A.
www.editions-la.com

The Sound Of L.A.
www.thesoundofla.com

Info Music
www.infomusic.fr

Delit Face
www.DelitFace.com

L.A. Unlimited
www.launlimitedinc.com

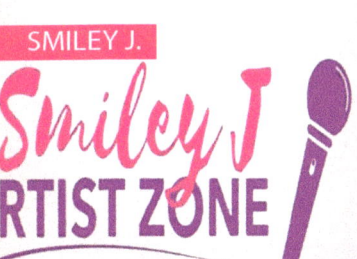

THE QUEEN OF THE BEST PODCAST FOR INDEPENDENT MUSIC ARTISTS

SMILEY J.

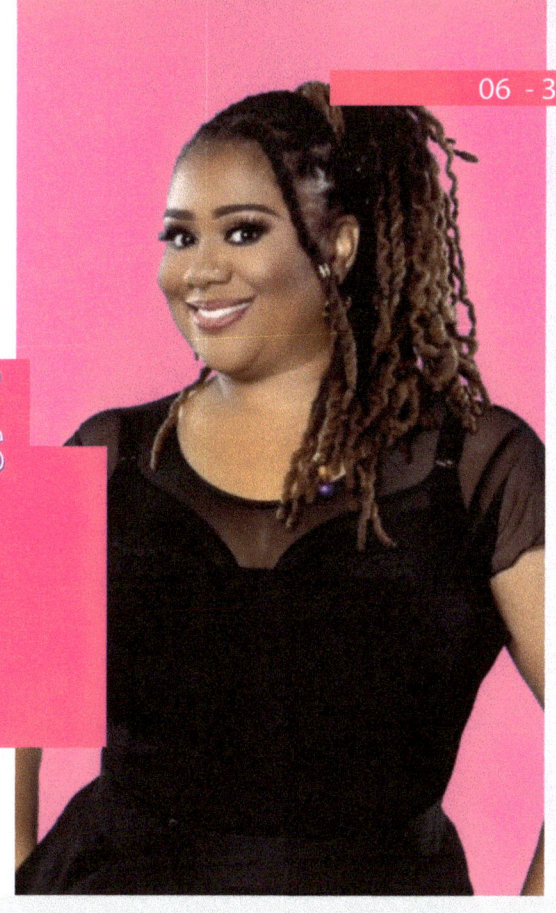

In the music fraternity today, there is a high rise in the number of independent musicians that have decided to independently release their music as opposed to the common use of commercial record labels or their subsidiaries. Some of these artists have also given up on the idea of being discovered.

A creative mind – Smiley J of "The Smiley J – Artist Zone" has created an amazing platform focused largely on independent musicians, their music, and upcoming events. "The Smiley J – Artist Zone" dropped as a podcast; a space dedicated to independent artists on which they are featured as guests to talk about their latest and upcoming projects in order to grow a wider fanbase among the many listeners of the podcast. The queen of the best podcast, "Smiley J," came up with this idea, and became the first host to an entirely independent artists' audio cast. Some independent artists that have already been featured on her podcast include; Selina Albright, singer and songwriter Eric Roberson, and many more others.

As a great listener and lover of a wider scope of music genres, Smiley J holds just one simple criterion for every guest on her podcast; "You must be an independent artist with music available for purchase on major music streaming platforms." Her platform is a great opportunity for every independent artist looking for more exposure to build a solid fanbase.
Podcasting in general has increasingly become popular in the world today. As opposed to actual radio show programs, many listeners are shifting habits and listening more to recorded and live podcasts. This is depicted in the increasing number of podcast listeners which was estimated at 120 million listeners in the USA as of 2021 with forecasts suggesting a further hike in the coming years.
"The Smiley J – Artist Zone" is a medium which should be embraced by every independent artist.

Together with the host, Smiley J, guests should anticipate a cool and fun conversation about their music journey, upcoming performances, and all other interesting areas of their music career. Because of the limited or no chance to sell their music to a considerably large number of listeners, independent artists have a chance with Smiley J's show to create a shortcut that would help them extend their music to a wider fanbase. This can be achieved through increased online streams and downloads on your music platforms, as long as you have what it takes to hold the listeners' attention.
For any new listeners or independent artists that would love to be featured on this podcast, be sure to tune in on your favourite music streaming or podcast platform every Thursday, at 7 PM, ET. Link to listen to the podcast; https://thesmileyjartistzone.podbean.com/.
Connect and stay in touch with the host Smiley J through her social media pages;
Instagram: @smileyj_artistzone
Facebook: The Smiley J Artist Zone
YouTube: The Smiley J Artist Zone
Email: TheSmileyJArtistZone@gmail.com

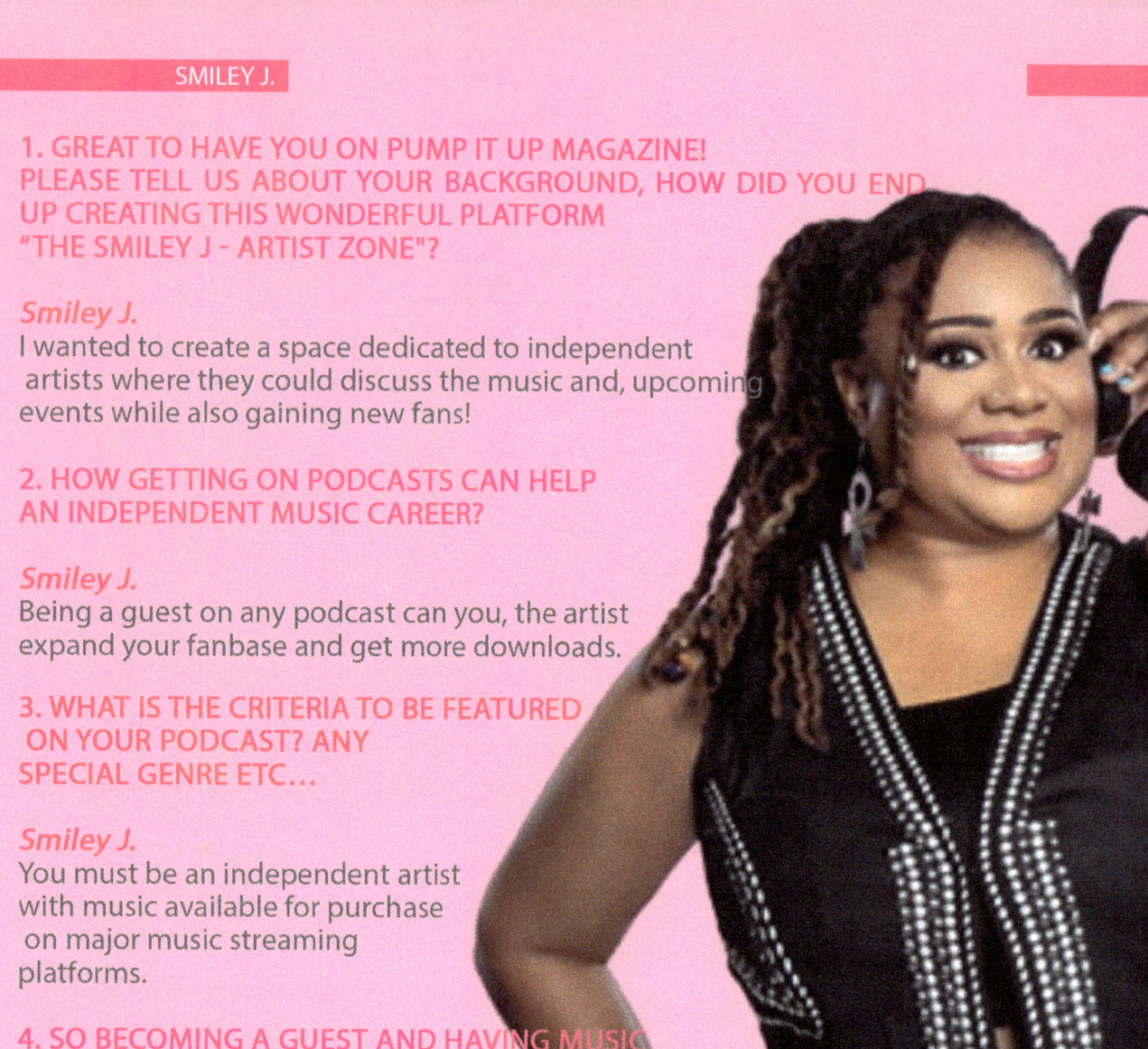

1. GREAT TO HAVE YOU ON PUMP IT UP MAGAZINE! PLEASE TELL US ABOUT YOUR BACKGROUND, HOW DID YOU END UP CREATING THIS WONDERFUL PLATFORM "THE SMILEY J - ARTIST ZONE"?

Smiley J.
I wanted to create a space dedicated to independent artists where they could discuss the music and, upcoming events while also gaining new fans!

2. HOW GETTING ON PODCASTS CAN HELP AN INDEPENDENT MUSIC CAREER?

Smiley J.
Being a guest on any podcast can you, the artist expand your fanbase and get more downloads.

3. WHAT IS THE CRITERIA TO BE FEATURED ON YOUR PODCAST? ANY SPECIAL GENRE ETC…

Smiley J.
You must be an independent artist with music available for purchase on major music streaming platforms.

4. SO BECOMING A GUEST AND HAVING MUSIC FEATURED ON YOUR ESTABLISHED PODCAST IS A GREAT OPPORTUNITY FOR INDEPENDENT ARTISTS WHO ARE LOOKING FOR MORE EXPOSURE TO BUILD A SOLID FANBASE. ANY ADVICE ON HOW THEY CAN PREPARE FOR THAT MOMENT?

Smiley J.
Yes, guests should be open to having cool, fun conversations about their music journey, upcoming performances, and some other fun stuff!

5. WHO ARE YOUR BIGGEST MUSICAL INFLUENCES? AND ANY PARTICULAR ARTIST/BAND YOU WOULD LIKE TO HAVE ON YOUR SHOW IN THE FUTURE?

Smiley J.
I listen to a lot of music from Jazz to Reggae and everything in between. I really just love music! I love songs with good lyrics it could be romantic, edgy, poetic, or political.
I love Sade, Bob Marley and, Lauryn Hill their music and lyrics just pulled me in! I would love to have Kellylee Evans who is from Canada and Liz Wright.

6. SO FAR, WHO HAS BEEN YOUR FAVORITE, OR MOST MEMORABLE GUEST ON THE SMILEY J - ARTIST ZONE"

Smiley J.
I really enjoyed Selina Albright she was a lot of fun great personality.

I also enjoyed Eric Roberson he is a great singer-songwriter, and he also gives a great concert! Super cool guy!

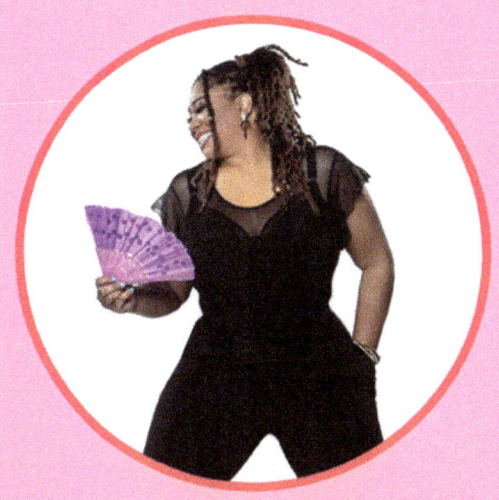

7. WHAT DOES THE FUTURE HOLD FOR THE SMILEY J - ARTIST ZONE"

Smiley J.
To feature more independent artists of various musical genres, to share their music journey, discuss new projects, upcoming performances and connect to their artists in a new way.
so they can introduce their new music and to my listeners

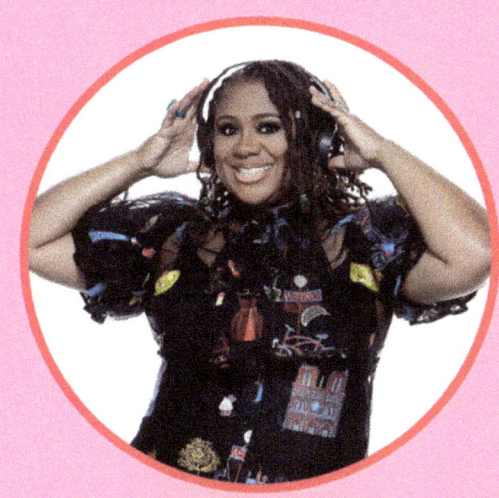

8. HOW CAN WE CONTACT YOU AND STAY UPDATED? ANY DIRECT LINK TO SUBSCRIBE TO YOUR NEWSLETTER?

IG smileyj_artistzone
FB; The Smiley J Artist Zone
https://thesmileyjartistzone.podbean.com

New listeners can listen to the show on their favorite music streaming platform.

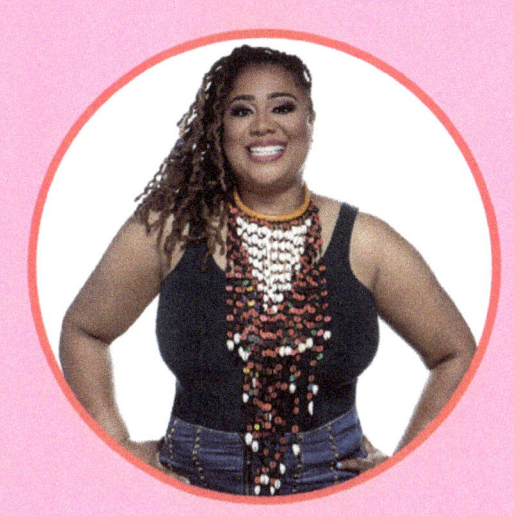

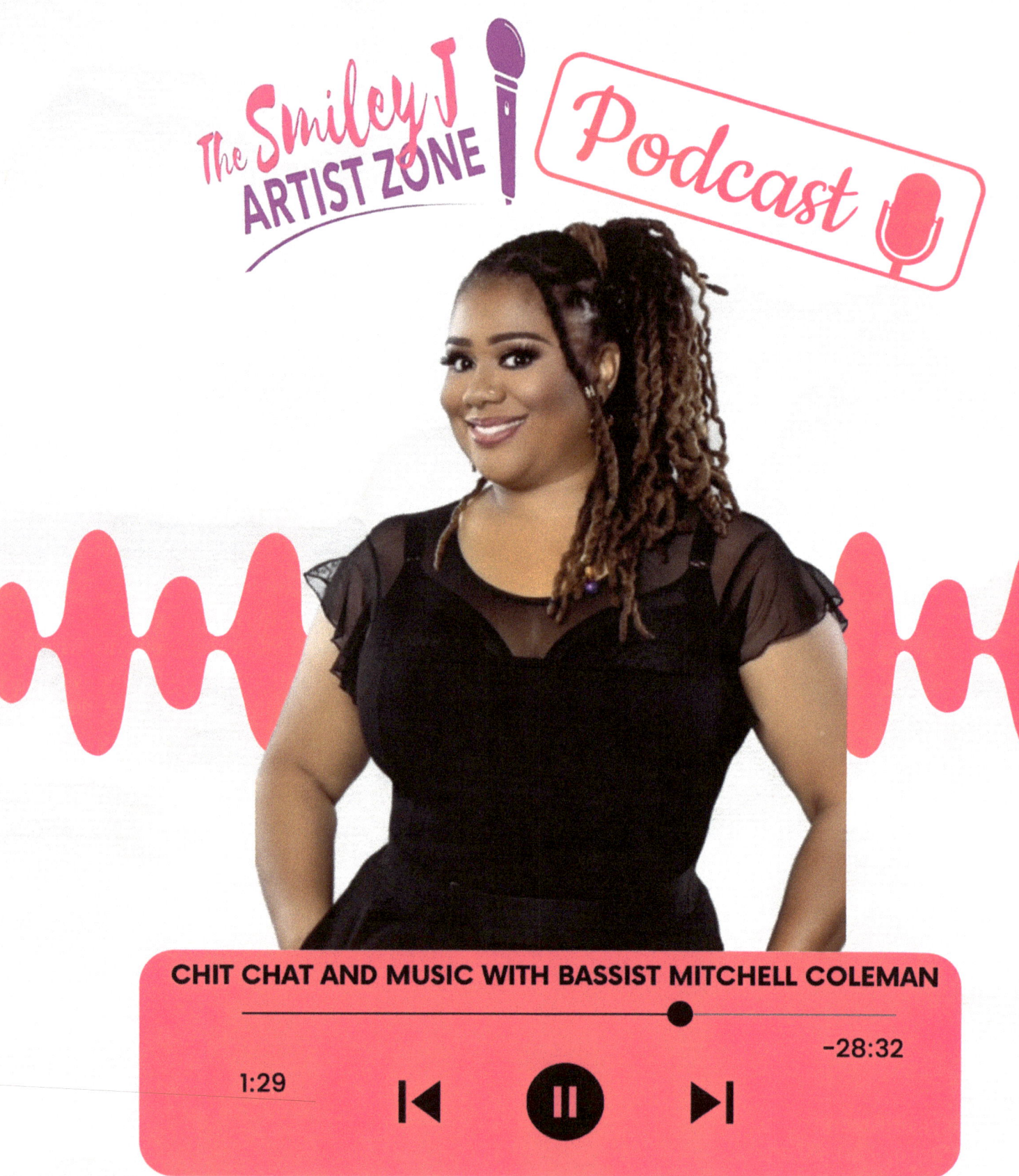

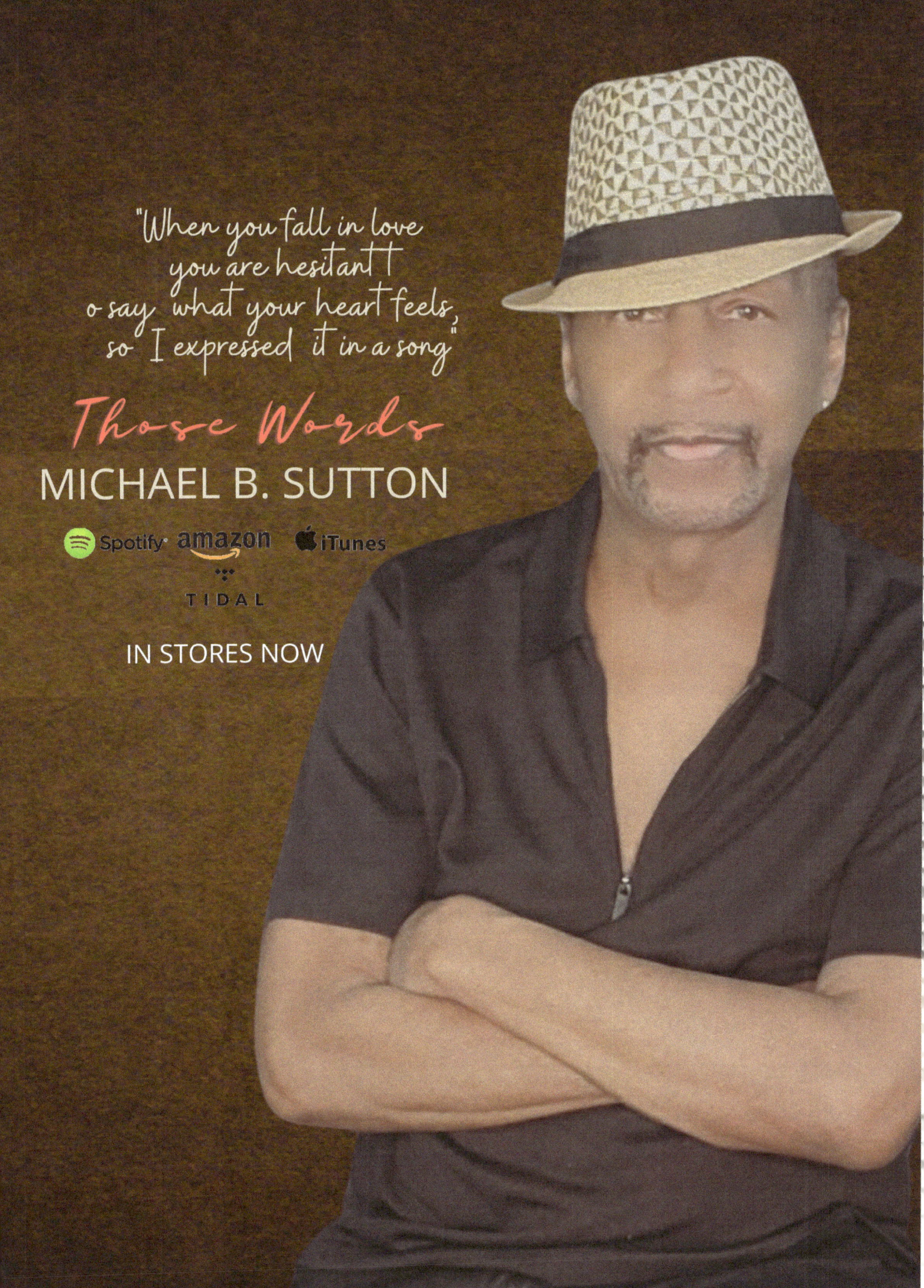

HOW GETTING ON PODCASTS CAN HELP YOUR MUSIC CAREER

1. BOOST YOUR ONLINE PRESENCE

One of the most significant benefits podcasting offers musicians is the ability to boost their online presence. Up-and-coming artists often lack the resources to launch an all-hands-on-deck campaign, even when they have something special to share with the world. Podcasting is one more avenue that provides a unique, convenient, and affordable way to highlight who you are as a person and as a musician.

There are several different podcast platforms that each reach millions of users on a daily basis. For instance, Apple's iTunes service has a podcast feature that is utilized by millions of listeners around the world every single day. This means that if you invest the time and energy into sharing a top-quality podcast to that network, you will have the chance of reaching an enormous audience by using a relatively simple and accessible method.

2. FAN BASE GROWTH

No matter how talented they may be, a musician is nothing without a fan base. It is essential that every working musician finds the time to grow their legion of followers, which is not easy to do. Podcasts are an often overlooked tool that can be used not only to spread the word about a new release or tell a story, but to reach new audiences who might otherwise completely miss your art. If you're only promoting yourself, nobody is going to tune in, but if you can find a way to hook people in some other way, they may get to know you, and soon your music.

As your fan base grows, so do your chances of reaching the ears of local businesses or event coordinators who are looking for fresh new content.

3. MUSIC PROMOTION

In addition to constantly creating new music, you must always be working hard to promote the tunes and albums you have already released. You can use podcasts, both your own and those run by others, to hype your latest single or perhaps to alert the world that you have a new full-length on the horizon.

The trick when it comes to spreading the word about your music is doing so in a way that interests people and doesn't come off as nothing more than a commercial.

4. NEW OPPORTUNITIES

Just as is the case with your music, you never know who is listening to you on the internet. Once you've put something out there for all to consume, it could reach anybody…and the more content (and the more different types of content) you release, the better your chances you touch someone who could help you reach new heights in your musical career.

Your podcast may be the thing that finds its way onto the phone of a promoter, an influencer, a booking agent or someone at a record label. If you do the medium right and give them something they're interested in, they may soon become a fan of your content…and then perhaps of your music itself.

Reach influencers, DJs, radio programmers and journalists with a full-scale promotional campaign.

5. NETWORKING

The internet has opened countless doors for everyone in the world to find like-minded individuals who work in their industries or share the same interests to interact, get to know one another, and even collaborate. Launching your own podcast means you are now one of many artists who also participate in that medium, and thus you may quickly begin meeting people in that space as well.

Invite others in the music industry and podcasting space to join you on your program, and they may return the favor. That helps you reach their audience, who might not know you already, and you never know what will come of your newfound partnerships!

6. WHY SHOULD EVERY MUSICIAN USE PODCASTS?

The short answer to this question is…why not? Podcasting has been picking up steam since its introduction into the online world years ago, and as time has gone by, many companies have dedicated their resources to perfecting the podcast medium, making the technology more accessible and streamlined for newcomers and seasoned users alike.

This is important because it allows the user to have a powerful tool at their disposal for any project they wish to share with the world. Long before podcasts and the internet existed, artists and bands often relied on big-budget marketing campaigns and traditional promotional tools that were ruled by gatekeepers. Today, podcasting has made it easier to reach a broad audience in a matter of seconds.

Whether you're a solo artist or a member of a band, you need to grab the attention of as many fans as possible to stand out from the crowd. With a professional podcast, you can reach the audience you want while boosting your musical, artistic, and even your personal presence.

Want to talk more about promoting your upcoming single or album? Contact Smiley J
Email: TheSmileyJArtistZone@gmail.com
Website:
https://thesmileyjartistzone.podbean.com

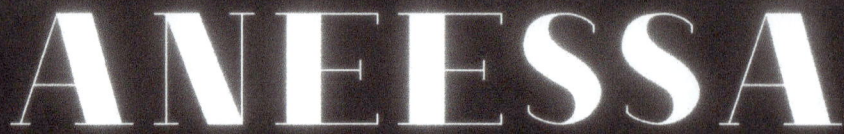

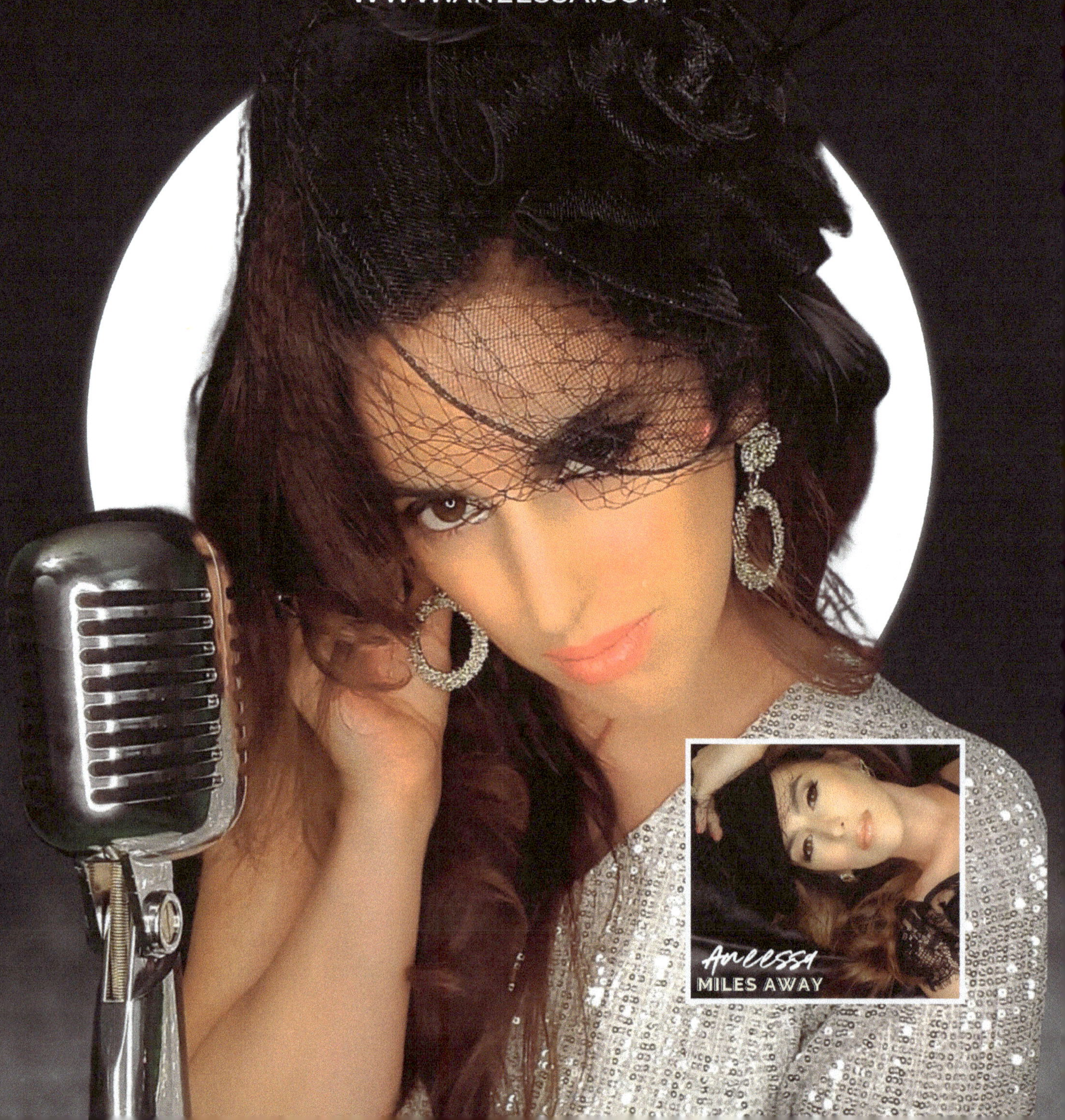

Editions L.A.

DIGITAL CREATIVE AGENCY

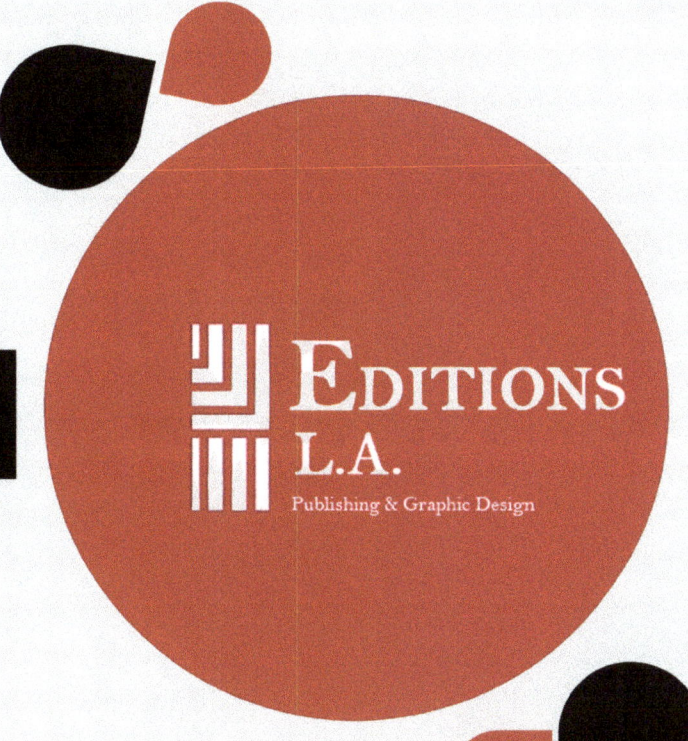

We Transform Your Vision Into Creative Results

Editions L.A. is a full-service agency based in Los Angeles. Our company is a collective of amazing people striving to build delightful services
We believe that is all about getting your message across clearly and with a "Wow!" thrown in for good measure.

Our Awesome Services

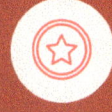

Branding

We build, style and tone your brand identity from the ground up.
We rebrand established bands, brands or businesses.

Merchandise Store
Website design and E-Commerce
Website updates

Digital Marketing

CD Cover | Banners | Logo design | Flyers | Brochures | Leaflets | Print ads | Magazine covers & artworks
Facebook / twitter / instagram / youtube artworks
| Book cover
Infographics | Icon Design |
| TshirtsProduct Labels | Presentation slides
Corporate graphics
Professional photo editing & enhancing
Redesign existing elements
YouTube Optimization and Monetization
Youtube Video Editing
Lyric Video and Advertising Design.

Publishing

BOOK COVER DESIGN
EBOOK FORMATTING SERVICES
and distribution on major platforms
(Amazon, Barnes & Nobles..)

Tell us about your dream and we will make it true!

Editions L.A.
7210 Jordan Avenue Suite B42, Canoga Park, California 91303, United States
info@edtions-la.com
Website: www.editions-la.com

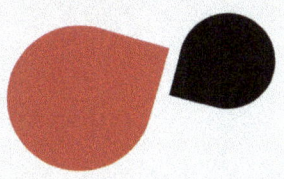

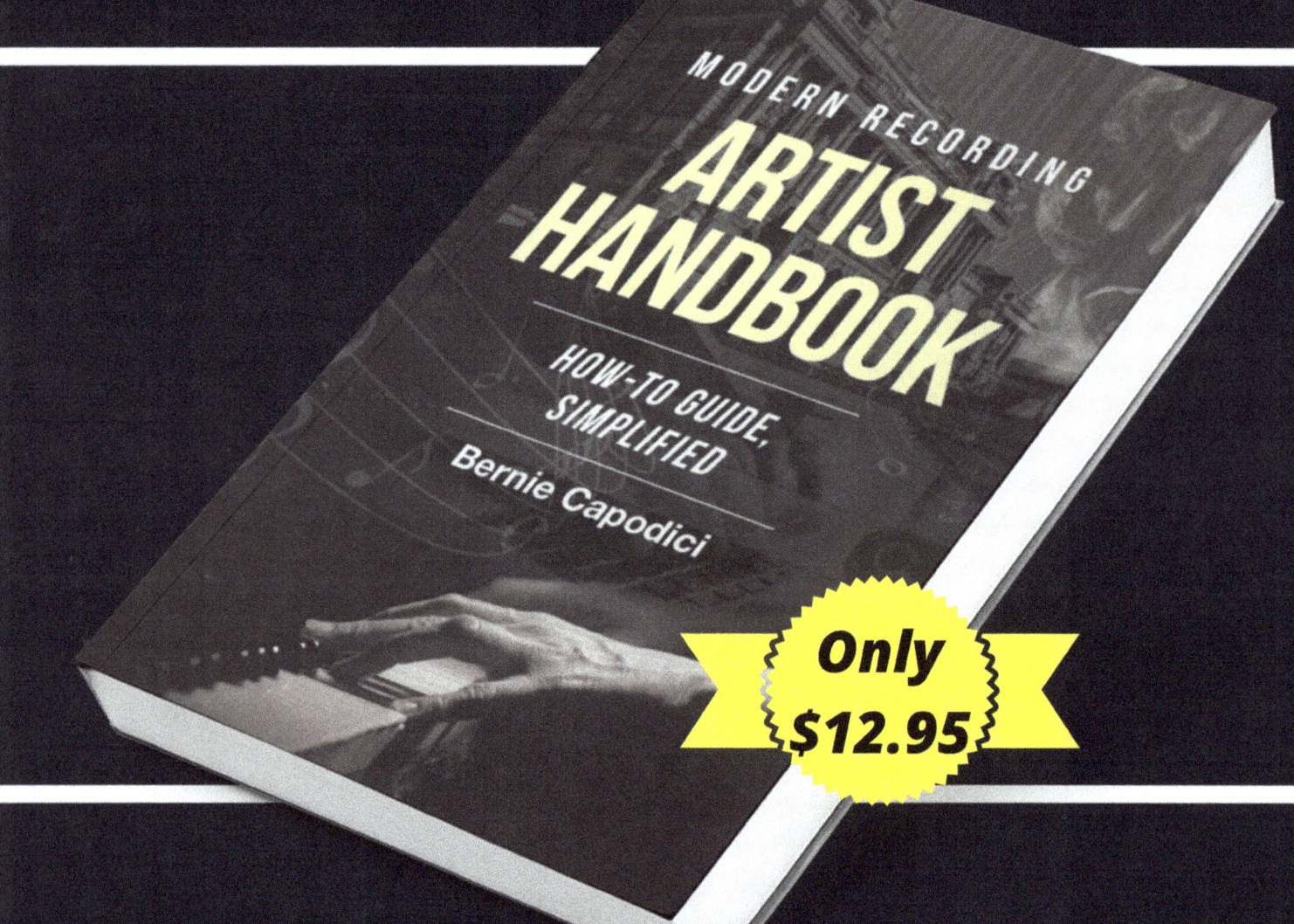

L.A. UNLIMITED

APPAREL REPRESENTATION
WITHOUT LIMITS...

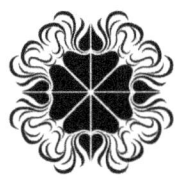

- Corporate Brand Representation
- Brand Identity & Management
- Brand Consulting
- Trade Show Preparation & Participation
- Trunk Shows
- Private Label Sales
- Production Sourcing

L.A. Unlimited & Associates
30765 Pacific Coast Hwy STE 443Malibu, CA 90265

310.882.6432
sales@launlimitedinc.com

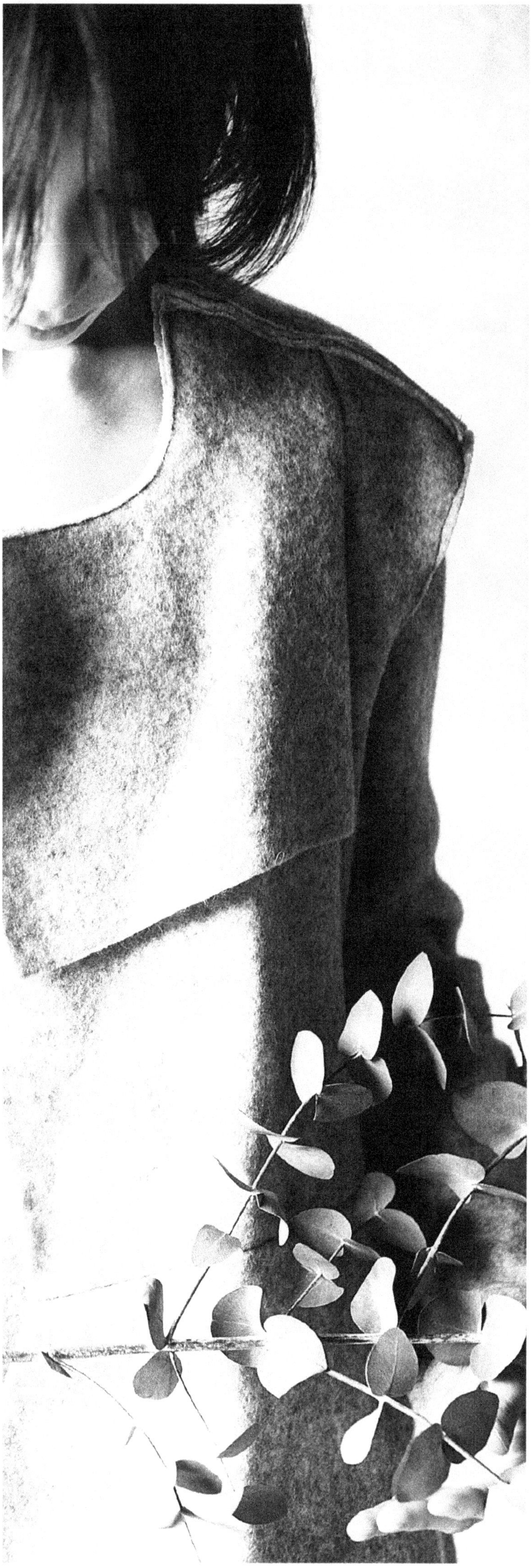

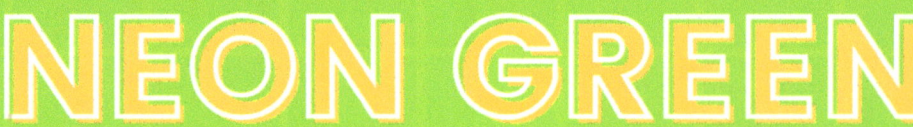

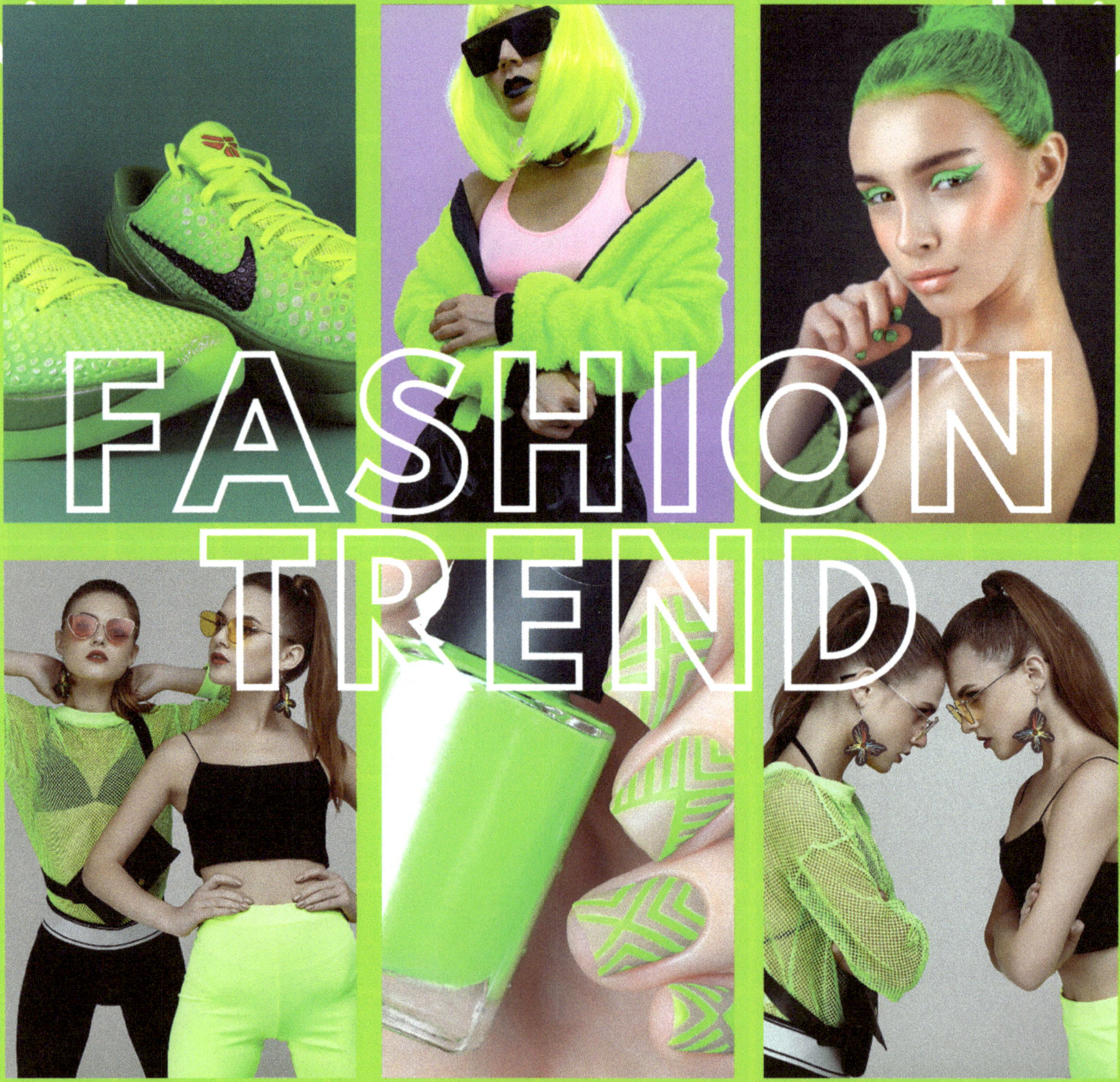

Fitness				18-34

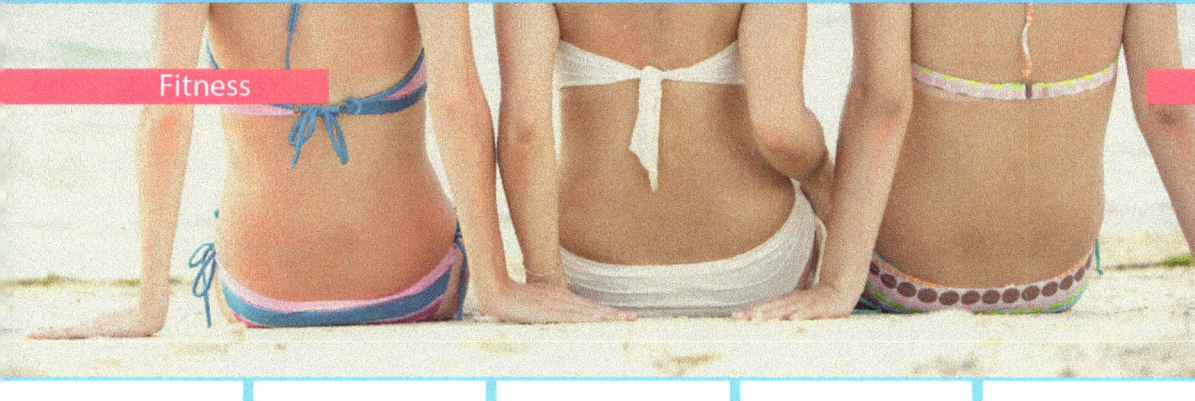
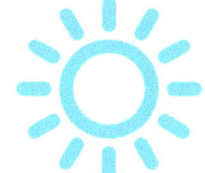

30 DAY BEACH BODY CHALLENGE

1	2	3	4	5
50 crunches 2x 60 second plank	50 crunches 2x 60 second plank	50 crunches 2x 60 second plank	50 crunches 2x 60 second plank	50 crunches 2x 60 second plank
6	**7**	**8**	**9**	**10**
50 crunches 2x 60 second plank	50 crunches 2x 60 second plank	50 crunches 2x 60 second plank	50 crunches 2x 60 second plank	50 crunches 2x 60 second plank
11	**12**	**13**	**14**	**15**
50 crunches 2x 60 second plank	50 crunches 2x 60 second plank	50 crunches 2x 60 second plank	50 crunches 2x 60 second plank	50 crunches 2x 60 second plank
16	**17**	**18**	**19**	**20**
50 crunches 2x 60 second plank	50 crunches 2x 60 second plank	50 crunches 2x 60 second plank	50 crunches 2x 60 second plank	50 crunches 2x 60 second plank
21	**22**	**23**	**24**	**25**
50 crunches 2x 60 second plank	50 crunches 2x 60 second plank	50 crunches 2x 60 second plank	50 crunches 2x 60 second plank	50 crunches 2x 60 second plank
26	**27**	**28**	**29**	**30**
50 crunches 2x 60 second plank	50 crunches 2x 60 second plank	50 crunches 2x 60 second plank	50 crunches 2x 60 second plank	50 crunches 2x 60 second plank

The 5-Days Love *Yourself Challenge*

Day 01 — Write Down What You Love About You

Day 02 — Create A Happiness Playlist

Day 03 — Cook Yourself A Nice Meal

Day 04 — Practice Self-Affirmation

Day 05 — Approach Your Problem With Mindfulness

@pumpitupmagazine

Wellness

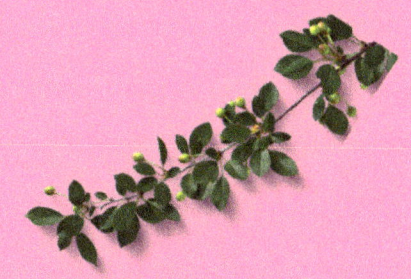

MENTAL DETOX

- Drink More Water
- Take A Relaxing Batch
- Set Goals For The Next Month
- Learn A New Hobby
- Find A New Podcast To Listen To
- Write Out A Bucket List
- Get 8 Hours Of Sleep
- Read A Favorite Book
- Do 30 Minutes Of Yoga

@pumpitupmagazine

How anxious are you?

OVER THE LAST 2 WEEKS, HOW OFTEN HAVE YOU BEEN BOTHERED BY THE FOLLOWING PROBLEMS	Not at all	Several days	More than half the days	Nearly every day
Feeling nervous, anxious or on edge	0	1	2	3
Not being able to stop or control worrying	0	1	2	3
Worrying too much about different things	0	1	2	3
Trouble relaxing	0	1	2	3
Feeling afraid, as if something awful might happen	0	1	2	3

What your total score means Your total score is a guide to how severe your anxiety disorder may be: •0 to 4 = mild anxiety •5 to 9 = moderate anxiety •10 to 14 = moderately severe anxiety •15 to 21 = severe anxiety If your score is 10 or higher, or if you feel that anxiety is affecting your daily life, call your doctor

HOW TO FIND A HOBBY IN ADULT AGE

It can often seem as though children have lots of hobbies – something for every day of the week (and sometimes twice) – but as they get older, those hobbies fade away. They become busier with their schoolwork, college, careers, friends, and families, and by the time they are fully grown adults, they don't have many interests left. They might not have any hobbies at all.

Yet having hobbies has been shown to be good for your mental and physical health, and they are great ways to discover more about yourself, keep fit (depending on the hobby, of course), meet other people, and so on.

If you're an adult looking for a new hobby, how can you even begin your search? Read on for some useful hints and tips.

THINK BACK

To begin with, the easiest option when it comes to thinking up a new hobby to enjoy as an adult is not to think of something new at all. Instead, think back to when you were a child. What did you use to enjoy then? Would you still enjoy it now? No matter what it was, whether it was painting, playing on a piano keyboard, martial arts, making clothes for dolls, reading adventure stories, or anything else, if it's something that you would like to get back into and that you would feel good about doing, why not do it?

Starting in this way doesn't have to be the end of your hobby search, but it is something that will help you focus your mind more directly. Plus, if there were hobbies you loved as a child, but that wouldn't work today, is there a more grownup version? Ideas can be adapted and changed, but you need to have those ideas in the first place.

ASK YOUR FRIENDS AND FAMILY

Asking your friends and family for advice and recommendations for anything you need to know more about in life is a good idea. You'll get honest, unbiased reviews about everything from the best local grocery store to the best place to buy fuel to the best tradesman to fix a leaking faucet. You do this without even thinking about it, so why not do it to find out about hobbies as well?

Of course, you might already know what they are into and enjoy doing in their spare time, and if any of those activities interests you, you can ask them for more information – people love to talk about their hobbies, and they will be more than happy to fill you in on how to get started.

Even if you don't want to join in with any of their hobbies, asking for recommendations is still a good idea. You might find out about things you never knew about before, which can open up many new opportunities and possibilities.

WHAT'S HAPPENING AROUND YOU?

If nothing comes to mind and there is nothing you are especially interested in, it can be easy to think there are no hobbies you would enjoy. However, there will always be something; you just need to know where to look.
Using social media is a good idea. You can join a group linked to your local area, and you'll immediately see all kinds of different activities being advertised. If you make it a rule to try something before you dismiss it altogether, especially if there is a free trial, you could get involved in many different local activities and find something you truly love.

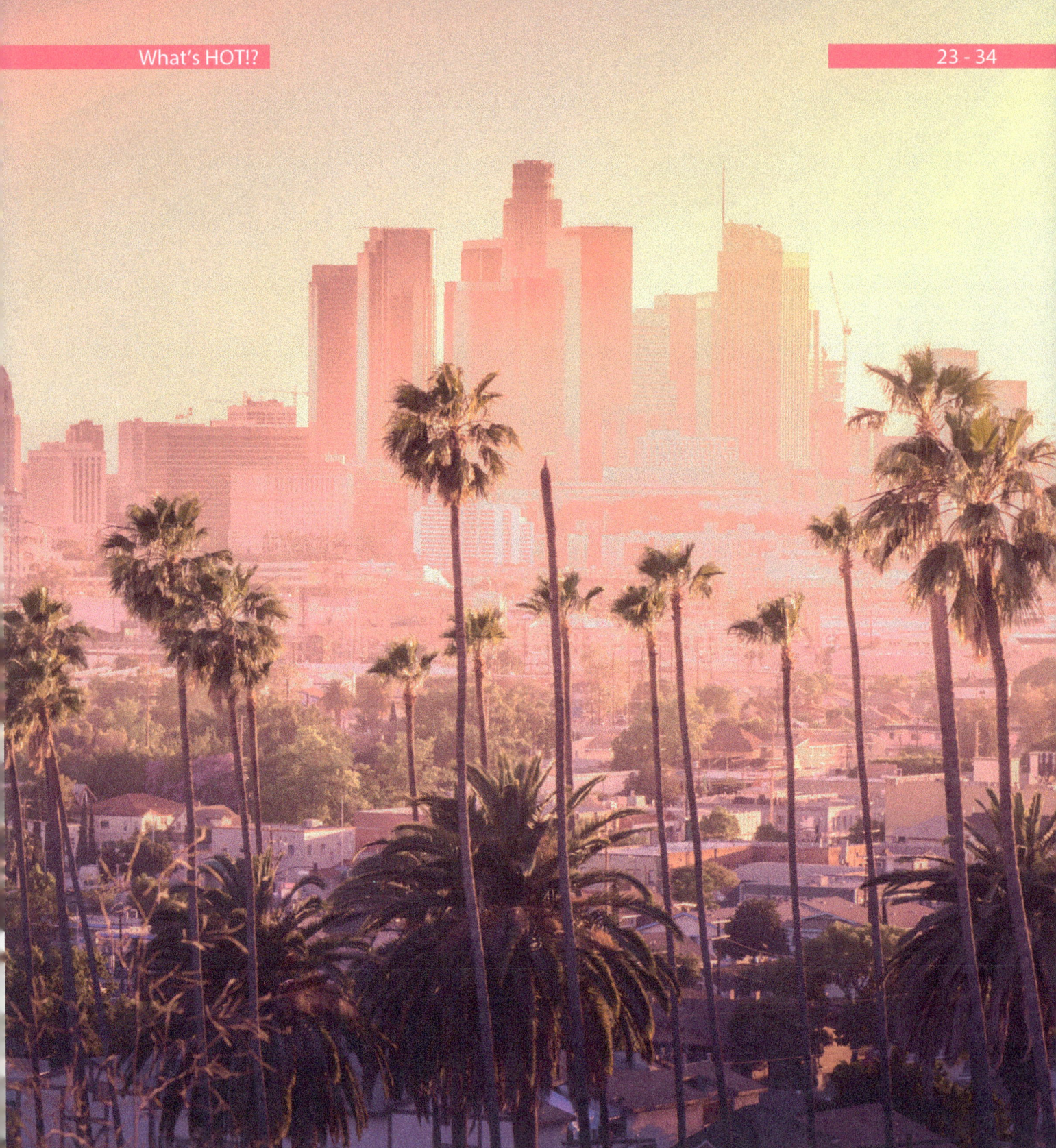

BEST THINGS TO DO IN

LOS ANGELES

What's HOT!?

BEST THINGS TO DO IN LOS ANGELES

Los Angeles has an exhaustive array of things to do. If you're a film buff, vintage Hollywood is a must-see. Some classic attractions in the area include TCL Chinese Theatre and the Hollywood Walk of Fame, and Paramount Pictures Studios, the only television and film studio left in Hollywood. For a taste of stardom, window-shop along Rodeo Drive or cruise Sunset Boulevard. There are also a plethora of shorelines to choose from, including Venice Beach, Zuma Beach and the Santa Monica Pier and Beach. Arts lovers will want to see a show at Walt Disney Concert Hall or swing by Los Angeles County Museum of Art to admire its collection. If you aren't sure where to start, a daylong guided tour of the city is a great way to orient yourself. And after exploring all LA has to offer, consider taking a daytrip south to Anaheim-Disneyland.

GRIFFITH OBSERVATORY AND GRIFFITH PARK
ADDRESS: 2800 E. OBSERVATORY ROAD

Griffith Observatory sits on the south face of Mount Hollywood and overlooks the Los Angeles basin. Its location gives visitors impressive views of the surrounding area, which many rave about. But there's more than just a pretty photo-op here. The observatory hosts fascinating exhibitions and features a top-notch planetarium.

SANTA MONICA PIER AND BEACH
ADDRESS: 200 SANTA MONICA PIER

Just west of downtown Los Angeles, Santa Monica contains one of the most legendary beach scenes in the United States. Santa Monica also boasts an abundance of great restaurants and excellent nightlife spots. The 3 miles of shoreline are renowned as some of the best in the area thanks to the soft sands, ideal weather and bevy of attractions. "State Beach," as it's known, has over 200 days of sunshine a year and acted as the backdrop for the popular television series "Baywatch."

HOLLYWOOD WALK OF FAME AND TCL CHINESE THEATRE
ADDRESS: 6925 HOLLYWOOD BLVD.

One of Hollywood's most iconic and memorable sites, the TCL Chinese Theatre (originally Grauman's Chinese Theatre) opened in 1927 and represents the excess of Hollywood's Golden Age. You can tour the theater for $18 (kids tour tickets cost $8 and senior tickets are $14 each); tours are offered from 10:15 a.m. to 7 p.m. every day except Monday

THE ORIGINAL FARMERS MARKET AND THE GROVE
ADDRESS: 6333 W. THIRD ST.

Sitting south of West Hollywood is one of LA's most beloved landmarks: The Original Farmers Market. Founded in 1934, this cream-colored facility reels in both residents and tourists with the promise of fresh produce and the aroma of ready-to-eat snacks

SUNSET BOULEVARD
ADDRESS: SUNSET BOULEVARD

One of the most iconic thoroughfares in the United States, Sunset Boulevard continues to live up to its legends. In the old days, it represented the classic and glamorous Hollywood lifestyle and became the setting of several famous films, including the obvious classic "Sunset Boulevard." Today, the palm-lined street (which connects downtown LA to Hollywood, Beverly Hills and the Pacific Coast Highway) retains its cinematic appeal, and the Sunset Strip portion has become a popular nightlife spot. The strip is also home to many classic music venues, including the Rainbow Bar & Grill and The Roxy Theatre.

YOUR MUSIC CONSULTANT

"YOU BELIEVE, SO DO WE!"

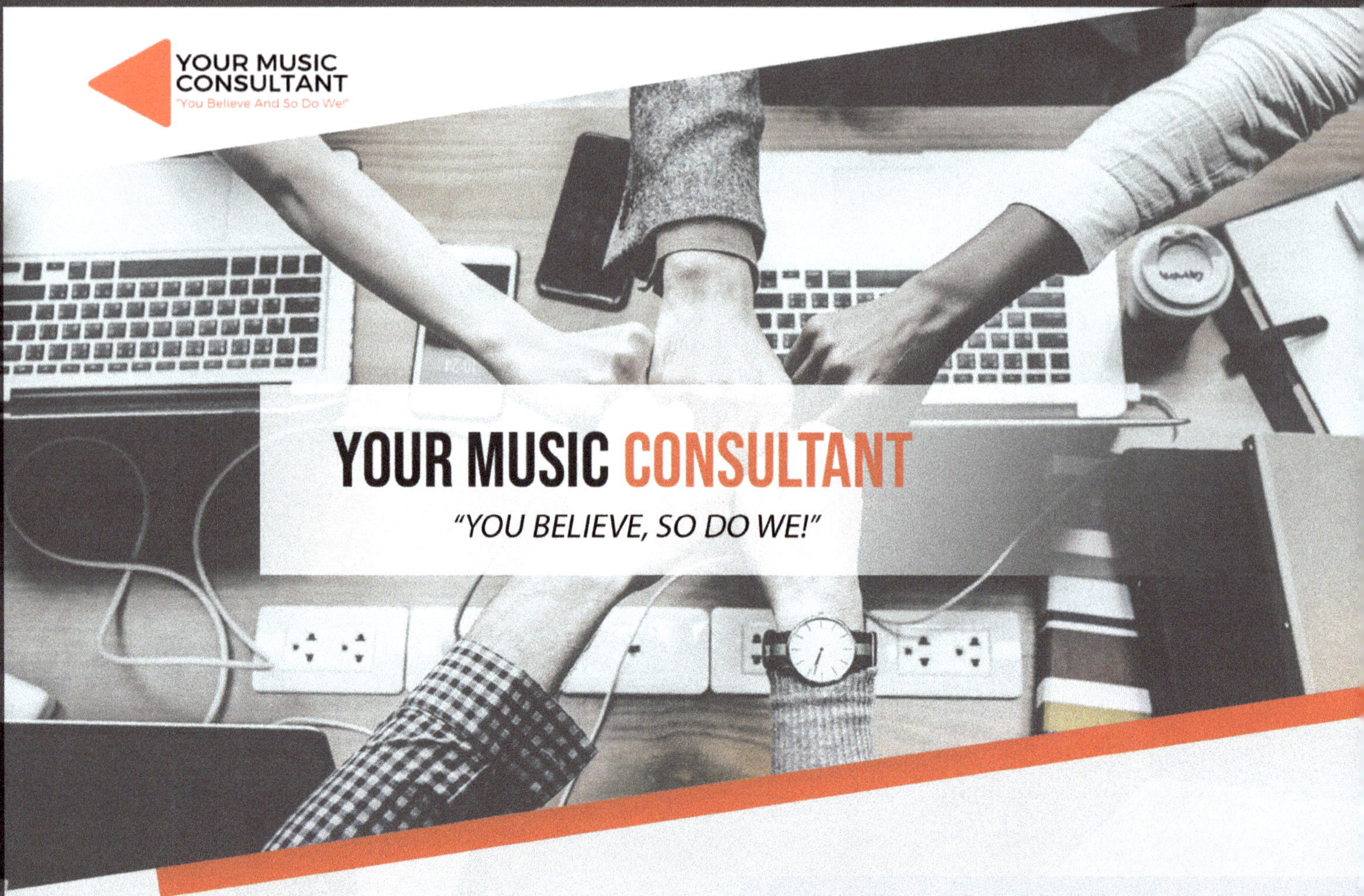

We Can Help You To Grow Your Business

We are a monthly based service, we put faith in artists who has major potential, believed in them, and who are willing to spend their time and own money to work with us in building a successful music career!

Digital Marketing Services

SOCIAL MEDIA - STREAMING SERVICES - MUSIC DISTRIBUTION - PRESS RELEASE - PRESS DISTRIBUTION - PR

Radio Airplay and TV Commercial

TERRESTRIAL AND DIGITAL RADIO CAMPAIGN AL GENRES EXCEPT HEAVY METAL - CABLE TV AND MAJOR NETWORK COMMERCIAL

Licensing & Booking

CONCERTS, LIVE MUSIC, EVENTS, CLUB NIGHTS - RED CARPETS - FOREIGN LICENSING AND SUBOPUBLISHING

Why Choose Us ?

3 DECADES OF MUSIC BUSINESS EXPERIENCE
Platinum and Gold Records
MOTOWN RECORDS
UNIVERSAL
SONY
CAPITOL RECORDS

WE WORKED WITH:

Kanye West - Jay Z - Stevie Wonder - Michael Jackson - Germaine Jackson - Smokey Robinson - Dionne Warwick - Cheryl Lynn - The Originals -

📞 **1 -818-514-0038**
(Ext. 1)
Monday - Friday / 9am to 6pm

FIND US :

www.YourMusicConsultant.com
30721 Russell Ranch Road Suite 140 Westlake Village, USA
Email : info@yourmusicconsultant.com

HOW TO COOK GREAT FOOD WITHOUT THE HASSLE

Cooking great food doesn't have to be a hassle. In fact, with the right tips and tricks, you can cook up a storm in your kitchen without breaking a sweat. This blog post is all about how to cook great food without the hassle – so read on for helpful tips and advice that will make your next meal time a breeze!

1) PLAN AHEAD

One of the best ways to avoid any kitchen hassle is to plan ahead. If you know what you're going to cook, you can easily gather all the ingredients and tools you need before getting started. This will save time and frustration later on. Another great way to plan ahead is to make a meal plan for the week. This will give you a variety of recipes to choose from, and it will help ensure that you have everything on hand when it's time to cook.

If you're feeling especially ambitious, why not try batch cooking? Batch cooking is where you cook multiple meals at once so that you have leftovers for later in the week. It's a great way to save time and energy in the kitchen.

2) USE THE RIGHT TOOLS

Having the right tools in your kitchen can make all the difference when it comes to cooking great food without the hassle. On the other hand, if you don't have the right tools, you might find yourself struggling to complete certain tasks, or you might wind up with a mess on your hands.

That's why it's crucial to invest in some quality kitchen tools. For example, an instant pot can be a lifesaver when it comes to quick and easy meals and will allow you to speed things up a notch, especially with recipes like these easy mashed potatoes in an instant pot. An air fryer is another excellent investment, as it allows you to cook delicious and healthy fried foods without using any oil. Of course, there are many other great kitchen tools out there – so be sure to do your research and find the ones that will work best for you.

3) COOK SIMPLE MEALS

One of the best ways to cook great food without the hassle is to keep things simple. If you're cooking a complicated dish, there's a good chance that something will go wrong. That's why it's often best to stick to simple recipes that are easy to follow. There are plenty of great simple recipes out there – and most of them can be made in under 30 minutes. So if you're looking for an easy way to avoid kitchen hassle, try cooking simple meals instead.

4) USE THE RIGHT TECHNIQUES

If you want to cook great food without the hassle, it's important to use the right techniques. If you're not sure how to do something, or if you're using the wrong approach, chances are things will go wrong in the kitchen.

That's why it's important to learn as much as you can about cooking techniques. There are plenty of great resources out there, such as cooking blogs, cooking classes, and even online tutorials. Once you learn the basics, you'll be able to apply them to any recipe – and that means less hassle for you in the kitchen.

Cooking great food doesn't have to be a hassle. With these helpful tips, you can breeze through your next meal time without any problems. So don't wait – start cooking up a storm in your kitchen today

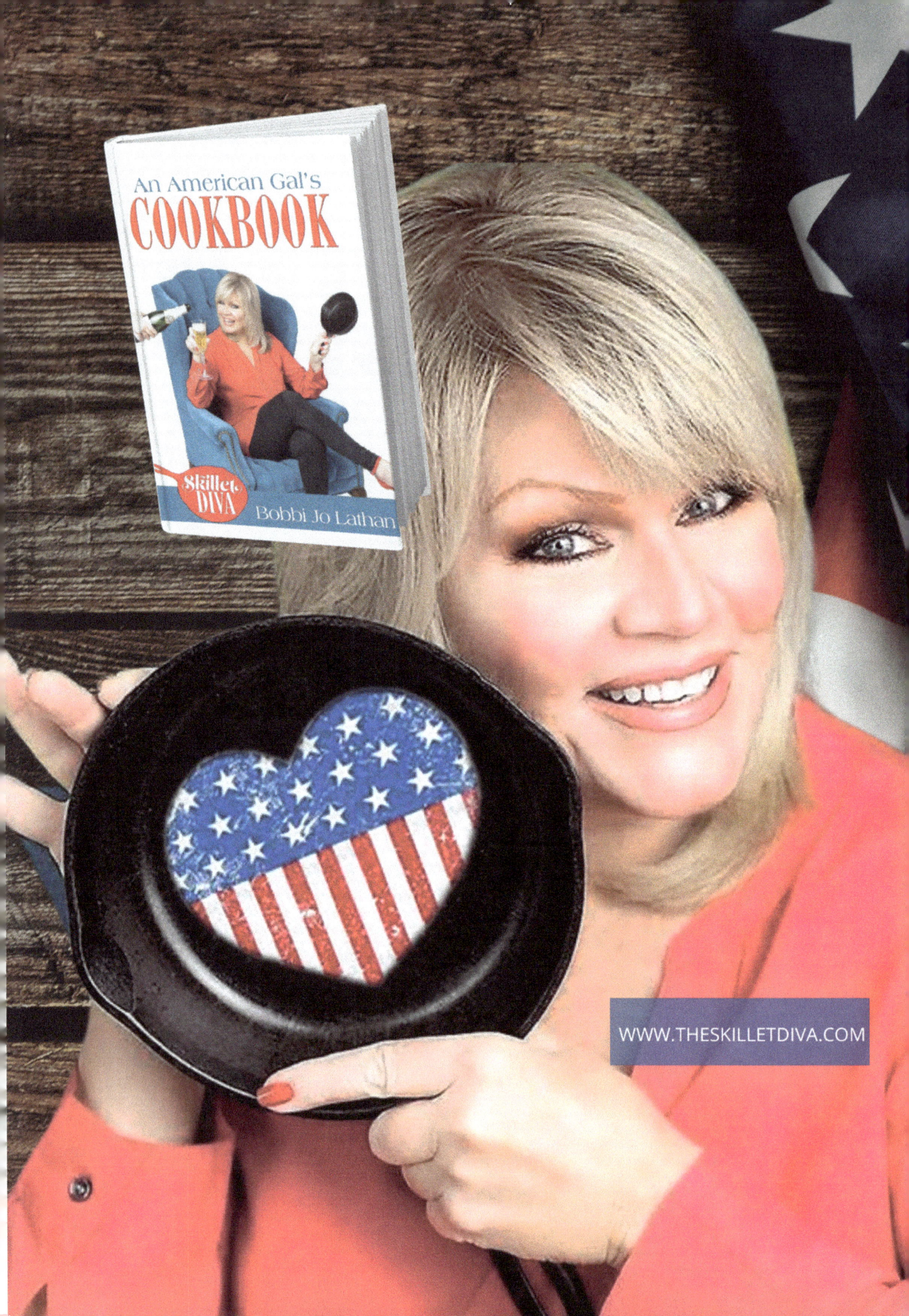

GAIN CONTROL OF YOUR SUBSCONSCIOUS MIND!

HYPNOTHERAPIST

Nader Hanna

818.445.1646

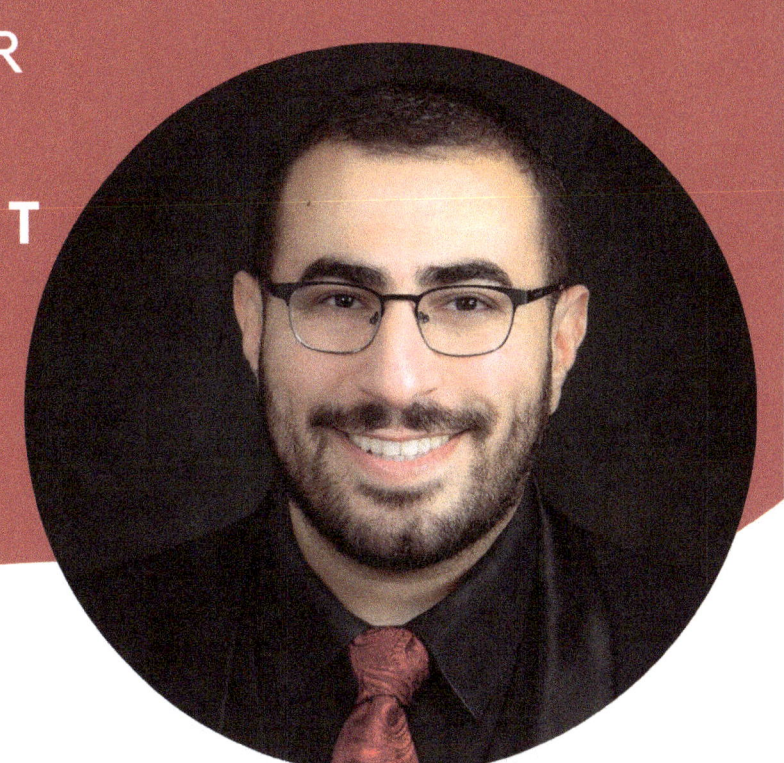

ABOUT

Nader's professionalism, warmth and flexibility coupled with his unique skills make him the perfect hypnotherapist to help you succeed in the positive changes in your life you have been dreaming of!

This Master Hypnotist is known for his mind-bending feats of ESP and hypnosis which he has displayed impressively while performing in shows for big names like John Landis, Joe Dante, Tippi Hedren, and at corporate events for companies such as NBC Universal.

HYPNOSIS WILL HELP YOU WITH

- **FEARS & PHOBIAS**
- **ANXIETY**
- **SPORTS PERFORMANCE**
- **FITNESS**
- **STOP SMOKING**

www.themasterhypnotist.com
www.themastermentalist.com

Los Angeles, California

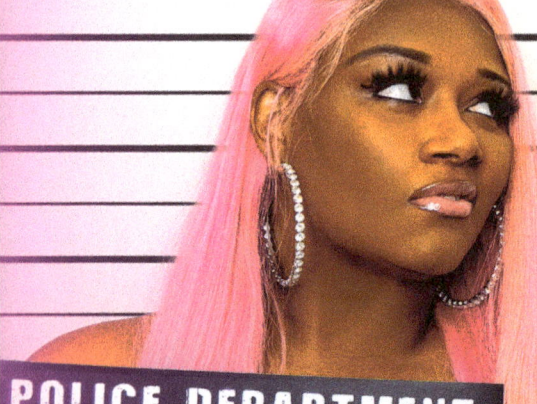

BEST INDIE MOVIES

There's no doubt about it: 2022 is looking to be a corker for films in terms of Hollywood big-hitters alone (The Batman, come at us). But when you delve into the gem-filled mine that is indie cinema, that's when you're bound to discover something unforgettable: a quiet, simmering masterpiece for the ages, let's say.
Year in, year out, Sundance Film Festival remains our go-to for all the best indie films to look out for and this year was certainly no exception, with its second virtual edition throwing up coruscating titles that have us cinephiles foaming at the mouth.

1. EMILY THE CRIMINAL

Everything Aubrey Plaza touches turns to gold – and this bleak, highly relatable crime thriller is at the top of our watch list. Emily's dreams of being an artist have amounted to nothing more than a stressful waitressing job to make ends meet and mounting student loan debt. It's no surprise she jumps at an opportunity to earn some quick cash; the only thing is, it's technically credit card fraud. But it's easy and only temporary, right? How far is she willing to go

2. FRESH

You'll remember Daisy Edgar-Jones from beloved sob-fest Normal People. The Irish actress is back, alongside Pam & Tommy's Sebastian Stan, navigating the dark side of modern dating. A pitch-black cocktail of social commentary and horror, we meet single woman Noa, who believes she's met her Prince Charming on a dating app: reconstructive surgeon Steve. When he invites her on a weekend away, she realises he's not all cookies and cream, and that's when the gore starts. He's a surgeon – you might be able to guess the rest

3. PHOENIX RISING

Evan Rachel Wood has been commendably brave for going public with her experiences of sexual assault and abuse at the hands of Marilyn Manson – and this gruelling, two-part HBO documentary sees the actress tell her story in full. It's certainly not an easy watch but delves into Wood's inspiring creation of the Phoenix Act, which understands that survivors of domestic violence need time to break the cycle and extends the statute of limitations on domestic violence felonies from three to five years.

4. GOOD LUCK TO YOU, LEO GRANDE

Nancy Stokes (queen Emma Thompson) is a lonely widow and retired schoolteacher yearning for some human connection and, well, sex. So she hires a sex worker for an afternoon of fun in an upmarket Norwich hotel room. It sounds cringe and crass but the result is a surprisingly tender comedy with a lot of things to say about sensuality, ageing and keeping the fire inside us alive.

5. MASTER

Take a prestigious, historically white university built in the shadow of the Salem witch trials, add three new Black students trying to survive the semester and you'll get Master – a thriller that certainly tips into the supernatural. Starring Regina Hall as longtime faculty member Gail, it ramps up the dread with stares, microaggressions and, later, straight-up racist vitriol. The horror is that the horror isn't too far removed from reality. It's a harrowing watch with Get Out vibes for sure.

3 WORDS YOU SEE
= PERSONALITY TRAITS

A	C	K	F	B	A	K
V	U	I	N	Y	M	H
B	O	N	S	Q	B	O
A	M	D	R	N	I	N
S	I	N	C	E	R	E
H	X	S	A	M	I	S
F	U	N	N	Y	O	T
U	O	S	Y	K	U	A
L	A	Z	Y	L	S	C

Awareness

HOBBIES TO REDUCE ANXIETY

Los Angeles has an exhaustive array of things to do. If you're a film buff, vintage Hollywood is a must-see. Some classic attractions in the area include TCL Chinese Theatre and the Hollywood Walk of Fame, and Paramount Pictures Studios, the only television and film studio left in Hollywood. For a taste of stardom, window-shop along Rodeo Drive or cruise Sunset Boulevard. There are also a plethora of shorelines to choose from, including Venice Beach, Zuma Beach and the Santa Monica Pier and Beach. Arts lovers will want to see a show at Walt Disney Concert Hall or swing by Los Angeles County Museum of Art to admire its collection. If you aren't sure where to start, a daylong guided tour of the city is a great way to orient yourself. And after exploring all LA has to offer, consider taking a daytrip south to Anaheim-Disneyland.

1. PLAYING MUSICAL INSTRUMENTS OR SINGING

Whether you are listening to music or playing an instrument, music is wonderful for stress relief and a great creative outlet. Playing a musical instrument helps develop your physical health, emotional well-being, and brings out your creative side. You don't have to be a professional musician to jam and enjoy good music.

2. JOURNAL WRITING

Writing can be therapeutic and a great release for all your mental worries. Writing in your free time helps process your emotions and thoughts.
Keeping a journal is easy. You just need a good journal and a pen. Journals are now sold with writing prompts to help you get started. If you are on a budget, a notebook will do. You can personalize it by labeling it with your name.

3. GARDENING

What is more relaxing than enjoying the warm sun and gazing at beautiful flowers? Whether you are growing flowers or vegetables, gardening is proven to relieve stress.
You can start by taking care of low-maintenance plants. If you don't have enough outdoor space for gardening, you can do indoor gardening by using pots or small garden beds.

4. PLAYING WITH PUZZLES

Mental rest doesn't necessarily mean your brain needs to stop doing mental work. Mental rest is basically doing something mentally engaging but not work-related.
Working with puzzles builds your mental strength. There are so many puzzle designs or pictures to choose from. If you decide to work on a big puzzle, you can have it framed when you're done with it. You can then hang it on your wall as decoration.

5. DRAWING AND COLORING

Drawing is a great way to process emotions and reduce stress. When your creative juices start to flow, you allow yourself to focus on yourself and you forget all your worries.
There are so many adult coloring books available with different designs and patterns you can choose from. Expressing your artistic abilities through coloring is a great way to reduce anxiety and alleviate stress.

6. DANCING

Turn up the music and dance to the beat. Dancing is a fun form of exercise and a fun physical activity. If you have been sitting in the office for hours, dancing is a good exercise with many health benefits..

HOBBIES TO REDUCE ANXIETY

Remember that your mental health matters

READING

Read a book you have been meaning to start.

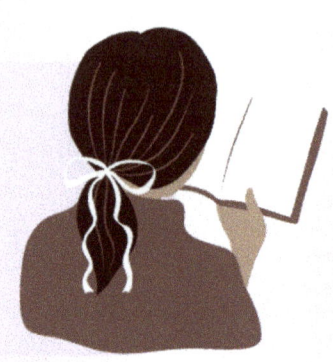

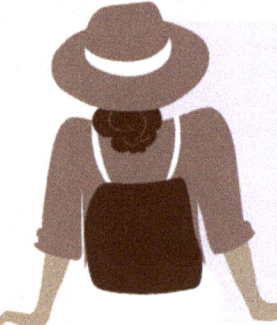

STAY ACTIVE

Find a hobby that keeps you active & encourages you to go outside.

MEDITATION

Spend time meditating for a few minutes daily to ease your thoughts.

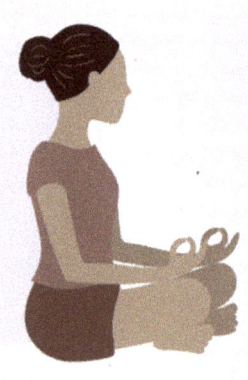

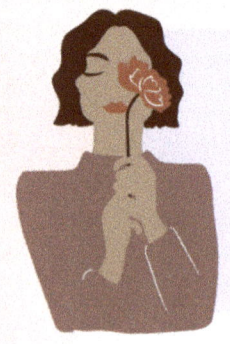

MINDFULNESS

Focus on paying attention to the present to relax your mind.

For more information, please visit:
www.pumpitupmagazine.com

www.ingramcontent.com/pod-product-compliance
Lightning Source LLC
Chambersburg PA
CBHW051810010526
44118CB00024BA/2821